CBD & Hemp Oil

Cannabis, Cannabinoids and the

Benefits of Medical Marijuana

By Aaron Hammond

Version 2.2

Published by HMPL Publishing at KDP

Get to know your publisher and his work at:

http://happyhealthygreen.life

A personal note from the writer

Since I have always been interested in cannabis and the medical benefits of marijuana, writing this book has been a pleasure. Since cannabis use has been on the rise, and there have been loads of positive results from research into cannabinoids, I am pleased to have the opportunity to share this information. I will teach you the basics of what cannabinoids do to our bodies and brains, and show you how this can be beneficial, including as a medicine.

I have been a recreational user of cannabis for more than ten years now, and when I had back problems last year I experienced first-hand the amazing pain-relieving effects of CBD and medical marijuana. I have tried to write this book as objectively as possible so that it is both unbiased and informative, but to be honest, with so many positive results and medical benefits, it is hard not to sell it as a miracle. I hope that in future, CBD and medical marijuana will continue to transform the world of medicine, and that legalization will make it possible for more and more people to enjoy their benefits.

If you have any questions during or after reading the book, please send me a personal email at hmpl.publishers@gmail.com

With kind regards,

Aaron Hammond

Disclaimer

The recipes provided in this report are for informational purposes only and are not intended to provide dietary advice. A medical practitioner should be consulted before making any changes in diet. Additionally, recipe cooking times may require adjustment depending on age and quality of appliances. Readers are strongly urged to take all precautions to ensure ingredients are of the highest quality.

The recipes and suggestions provided in this book are solely the opinion of the author. The author and publisher do not take any responsibility for any consequences that may result due to following the instructions provided in this book.

Bonus

Welcome to HMPL Publishing!

Let's start right away with an exclusive bonus made available only to HMPL subscribers. Want to get our book 'The best DIY THC & CBD recipes to prepare at home' for free? Go to: http://eepurl.com/cxpVZf

Subscribing to our newsletter will get you the latest THC- and CBD-recipes, interesting marijuana-related articles and a chance to win one of our upcoming books for absolutely free. With each release, we randomly select 5 subscribers that will get our book free of charge.

Want our free book, stay keen on medical breakthroughs and the various applications of cannabis? **Subscribe** to the HMPL Publishing newsletter and grab your free copy of 'The best DIY THC & CBD recipes to prepare at home'. All you have to do is enter your email address to get instant access.

We don't like spam and understand you don't like spam either. We'll email you no more than 2 times per week. Go to: http://eepurl.com/cxpVZf

You can also follow us on Facebook;
https://www.facebook.com/HMPLpublishing

Table of Contents

A personal note from the writer...3

Disclaimer..6

Bonus...7

The benefits of hemp and hemp oil 9

What do you know about CBD?.....................................16

Important medical message 18

What is CBD?...22

Cannabinoids and how they work 24

What does CBD do, exactly?..26

Medical uses and applications.......................................28

How you can use CBD 32

Dosing with CBD oil...35

How is CBD hemp oil used to create CBD products?.....37

Making your own CBD oil 38

Topical and edible recipes made with CBD oil..............48

CBD topical hand balm 49

CBD cookies...51

Bonus reminder 54

Thank you..55

Supportive research papers..56

The benefits of hemp and hemp oil

First off, let's talk about hemp, a plant that belongs to the *cannabis sativa* family. Hemp has been cultivated for thousands of years as a source of fibre, edible seeds, edible oil, lubricant, and fuel.

In industry, hemp is generally used to produce the industrial grade CBD-rich hemp oil and other CBD (cannabidiol) products. This should not be confused with the modern legal cannabis industry. The latter offers a wide variety of new strains that are rich in CBD and contain the least amount of THC possible. (THC, or tetrahydrocannabinol, is the chemical compound in cannabis responsible for the euphoric high.) Such strains are much more efficient than common hemp when it comes to CBD production. Nonetheless, the health and nutritional benefits of hemp itself are noteworthy. In regard to CBD, I would recommend using a cannabis strain that has been specifically bred to produce large quantities of CBD. In terms of efficiency, hemp cannot be compared to CBD-rich strains of cannabis, and large amounts of hemp are needed to produce CBD extracts. That said, you will often see products labelled CBD-rich hemp oil and tinctures. This is just to clear up any confusion that might be caused. In short, CBD-rich hemp products generally come from industrial-grade hemp.

Hemp is the industrial form of *cannabis sativa*. It contains only a small percentage of cannabinoids such as CBD and THC because (unlike cannabis) it is not grown as a drug. Hemp offers us many nutritional and health benefits, as well as clothing, rope and oil.

First, we will talk about hemp seeds and their benefits in our daily lives. Later, we will get into the specifics of hemp oil. More importantly, we will discuss the medicinal benefits of CBD and other cannabinoids derived from cannabis and hemp.

The benefits of hemp seeds

Those little hemp seeds are truly a gift of nature. They are the most nutritious seeds in the world, and offer us a complete protein. In fact, hemp seeds are known to have the most concentrated balance of proteins, essential fats, vitamins and enzymes. With their relative absence of sugar, starches and saturated fats, you could consider hemp seeds a potent superfood. They are one of the most potent foods available, supporting optimal health and well-being. Hemp seeds give us a broad spectrum of health benefits, including weight loss, increased and sustained energy, rapid recovery from disease or injury, lowered cholesterol and blood pressure, reduced inflammation, a better circulation and immune system, and natural blood sugar control.

Hemp seeds contain a perfect and natural blend of easily digested proteins. They also contain essential fatty acids such as Omega 3 & 6, antioxidants, amino acids, fiber, iron, zinc, carotene, phospholipids, phytosterols, vitamin B1, vitamin B2, vitamin B6, vitamin E, vitamin D, chlorophyll, calcium, magnesium, sulfur, copper, potassium, phosphorus, and enzymes. In them are all the amino acids essential to optimal health, including the rare Gamma Linolenic Acid (GLA). Every 100 grams of hemp seed provides 17+ grams of omega fats. That's enough to give you continuous energy throughout the day. Besides having all the benefits mentioned above, hemp seeds are:

-high in protein

-easy to digest

-suitable for people with allergies to nuts, gluten, lactose or sugar.

Essential fatty acids in hemp seeds

The oil in hemp seeds is broken down into 75-80 percent polyunsaturated fatty acids (the good fats) and only 9-11 percent of the less desirable saturated fatty acids. This makes hemp seed oil the most unsaturated oil that can be derived from plants. The essential fatty acids (EFAs) contained in hemp seed oil are not naturally produced by our bodies. Hence they must be obtained from the food we eat.

Having 78 percent of these essential fats, hemp oil is much better than soy oil (40 percent), canola oil (30 percent), olive oil (10 percent) or other oils. Omega 3 and Omega 6, the essential fatty acids, may reduce your incidence of cholesterol, blood pressure, coronary heart disease and stroke. Most health organizations suggest that the human body needs a 3 or 4:1 ratio of Omega 6 to Omega 3. Hemp seed is the only seed in which this ideal balance occurs naturally. Hemp oil contains more Omega 3 EFA components (19 percent) than are found in any fish or in most fish-oil supplements, or oils from flax, almonds, walnuts, soybeans or olives. In fact, the daily use of flax seed could lead to dangerous imbalances, since flax seed oil has a ratio of 1:4 of Omega 6 to Omega 3, instead of a healthy 4:1 ratio.

The essential fatty acids mentioned earlier help to produce energy in the human body. Without them, life is not even possible. But to be blunt, North Americans have a high dietary deficiency of EFAs because of all the processed foods and meats they eat.

In addition, extensive studies have shown that many common illnesses are related to deficiencies or imbalances of specific fatty acids in the body. Symptoms often spring from a lack of Omega 3 and Omega 6 fatty acids and their derivatives, the prostaglandins.

It has been proven in several clinical studies that dietary supplementation with EFAs or their metabolites (such as gamma-linolenic acid or GLA) will often prevent or even cure many illnesses and health conditions.

A natural source of energy

To put it simply, hemp seeds are about one-third oil and one-quarter protein —for cellular health and energy. Hemp seeds outshine most energy bars in that they provide energy in a better form, without sugar and saturated fats.

Four tablespoons of hemp seeds (42 g), enough to sprinkle on cereal, fruit, yogurt or salad, contain:

240 Kcal energy

15 grams of essential fats (11.4 g Omega 6 and 3.6 g Omega 3)

2.7 grams mono-unsaturated fat

2.1 grams saturated fat

15 grams of protein

2.5 grams of fiber

4.5 grams of carbohydrates

It should be noted that hemp seeds do not contain cholesterol.

Hemp protein

Hemp protein is also a complete source of all twenty known amino acids, including the nine essential amino acids (EAAs) which our bodies cannot produce. About 65 percent of the protein is made up of the globulin protein *edestin* which is found only in hemp seed. Edestin aids digestion, is relatively phosphorus-free, and is considered to be the backbone of the cell's DNA. The other one-third of hemp seed protein is *albumin*, another high-quality globulin protein, similar to that found in egg whites. Hemp protein has no tryspin inhibitors which block protein absorption, and none of the oligosaccharides that soy contains, which can cause stomach upsets and gas.

Hemp seeds provide a more digestible protein than meat, whole eggs, cheese, human milk, dairy milk, or any other high-protein food. They have a better spectrum of available proteins than soybeans, and lack the anti-nutritional factors of soybeans. They are an excellent protein product for everyone — mothers, babies, body builders, convalescents, and the elderly.

Hemp seed is an unsurpassed source of the whole spectrum of required proteins. It promotes vigorous cellular development, with diverse health benefits such as:

-Reduced cholesterol and blood pressure, thereby decreasing the risk of stroke

-Less of the inflammatory characteristics of many hundreds of diseases

-A more rapid recovery from disease, from radiation treatment, and from injury

-A more effective immune system, with reduced incidence of all types of disease

-Less inflammation in such conditions as arthritis, cardiovascular disease, psoriasis and even tuberculosis

-In diabetics, better circulation and less inflammation.

What do you know about CBD?

Now that you have learned what hemp can offer your health, we turn to *cannabis* and *cannabinoids*. First, let's be clear on our definitions. *Cannabis* is the species name for the entire marijuana plant. The term *cannabinoid* refers to one of a number of chemical compounds found within the plant. *Cannabidiol,* or CBD, is one of the most prevalent of these chemical compounds, but it is non-psychoactive, unlike the more famous molecule *tetrahydrocannabinol* or THC.

Earlier, we mentioned how hemp and cannabis were of the same family. *Hemp* is low in cannabinoids and is used in the food industry, while *cannabis* has been bred for its psychoactive properties. This difference is noticeable when it comes to the ratio of THC and CBD in these subspecies. Hemp has an industrial ratio of 0.2 percent THC, with slightly more CBD ingredients, whereas cannabis can have more than 30 percent of THC, and can be specifically bred to contain high CBD, up to 1:20, meaning 1 percent THC and 20 percent CBD.

As mentioned earlier, CBD is short for *cannabidiol.* It is found in the well-known and once illicit cannabis plant and in the legal industrial version of the plant called hemp. It is known that CBD has a lot to offer. But only recently have cannabis, THC and CBD received positive media attention, with their stigma as illegal, Schedule I drugs having been removed. The legalization of marijuana has become a trending topic over the last couple of years. Recently, 29 American states said 'yes' to the medical use of marijuana, while the recreational use of marijuana was approved in eight states across the USA.

But the USA is not the only player. The UK plans to legalize cannabis for medical use and Canada gave the green light for medical use back in June 2015. There has also been positive news from other countries in Europe and on the other side of the world. It seems the tide is changing for Australia, since the medical use of marijuana has been legal since November 2016.

Now that we are talking legal use, then, there is much information to be shared. Precisely what is CBD and how does it differ from THC? How does CBD work, and what are the positive and negative effects on your body and brain?

Important medical message

(This is about the medical use of CBD and its potentially harmful side-effects and interactions with regular medicine.)

As I am a firm believer in self-medication with CBD for many ailments that don't require the attention of a doctor or specialist, I do have to state the importance of the following message: If you have a serious condition such as epilepsy, cancer, COPD or other serious diseases or conditions where CBD and THC could have a significant medicinal value, I urge you to discuss this with your medical practitioner. Find out how CBD could interact with your current medicine, and how harmful side effects could be prevented.

Drugs that interact with cannabidiol

Below we list the types of drugs that are metabolized by cytochrome P450 and interact with cannabidiol. (Cytochrome P450 enzymes are primarily found in liver cells but are also located in cells throughout the body. These enzymes metabolize external substances, such as medications that are ingested, and internal substances, such as toxins that are formed within cells.) According to the Indiana University Department of Medicine, drugs known to be metabolized by the cytochrome P450 system include:

-steroids

-HMG CoA reductase inhibitors

-calcium channel blockers

-antihistamines

-prokinetics

-HIV antivirals

-immune modulators

-benzodiazepines

-anti-arrhythmias

-antibiotics

-anesthetics

-anti-psychotics

-anti-depressants

-anti-epileptics

-beta blockers

-PPIs (proton-pump inhibitors)

-NSAIDs (nonsteroidal anti-inflammatory drugs)

-angiotensin II blockers

-oral hypoglycemic agents

-sulfonylureas

Keep in mind that this list of drugs does not necessarily contain every from of medication that could potentially be affected by cannabidiol. Also note that not every medication in each of the categories listed will cause an interaction. For this reason, you should consult with a medical professional before taking any combination of drugs, as alternative medications or dosage adjustments may be required. If you are worried that your P450 enzyme system may not be functioning properly, physicians can test you to ensure that the medications you take are metabolizing as they should.

Regarding the recipe and method of extraction provided in this book, I cannot give you any medically approved indication of the required dosage. This is also something you should discuss with your medical practitioner, but I am aware that not everybody might be in a situation where this is possible. And some readers may have to deal with biased medical practitioners whose narrative does not include the use of medical cannabis and CBD.

For those who lack access to direct and unbiased medical advice or treatment, I will present safe and commonly accepted ways to administer and measure CBD. I will also give you advice from the heart. I want to provide information on this subject at an understandable level for everyone. This book is not a critically acclaimed science paper but a collection of important, researched and easy-to-understand items of information. At the end you will find a list of research papers and clinical trials that back up the information we provide.

Many people cannot pay for expensive, lab-tested CBD products with price indications like $700 for 3600mg of pure CBD. So I want to provide the information and methods that will enable them to procure their own medicine and apply it in different situations. In some places it may be illegal to buy them, but cannabis and CBD can be highly useful for various medicinal purposes.

In this book, I aim to provide scientifically-researched information for everyone, to focus on the most important effects of CBD, and to keep things simple. In my view, the use of cannabis, which is easily grown, made, measured and used by individuals, should not be held back by companies that are already trying to squeeze a buck out of every aspect of this medical breakthrough. Some people have no insurance coverage that would enable them to buy these products for themselves, but they need CBD and cannabis as medicine. They are the ones I want to help. As I mentioned earlier, the medicinal use of cannabis and CBD *can* have unwanted and harmful side effects in counteraction with regular pharmaceutical drugs. If that applies to you, I strongly recommend you get professional advice in these matters. Otherwise you use them at your own risk.

This book is written mainly at a basic level. I am currently working on several other books on cannabis-related subjects such as a DIY cannabis extraction guide, a guide to growing cannabis, cookbooks, and detailed books covering the science behind cannabis. Some of them will be written at a basic level also, because I want this information to be accessible, understandable and readable by everyone.

What is CBD?

As you read in the introduction, the term CBD is short for *cannabidiol*. This is a cannabinoid found in cannabis or hemp and is one of at least 115 active cannabinoids identified in cannabis. Cannabinoids are found in two species of cannabis—*cannabis sativa* and *cannabis indica*. While hemp is part of the same family as *cannabis sativa,* there is a significant difference in the THC/CBD levels between industrial cannabis and cannabis as a drug. The THC and CBD components of cannabis have been enhanced over the years, but hemp has stayed pretty much the same, being used for industrial production. So the cannabinoid components and levels of THC and CBD in hemp are notably lower.

2-[(1R,6R)-6-isopropenyl-3-methylcyclohex-2-en-1-yl]-5-pentylbenzene-1,3-diol2-[(1R,6R)-6-isopropenyl-3-methylcyclohex-2-en-1-yl]-5-pentylbenzene-1,3-diol

In cannabis and cannabinoids there are two major phytocannabinoids. One is called *cannabidiol,* or CBD for short. The other is called *tetrahydrocannabinol,* or THC. THC is the primary psychoactive compound found in cannabis, and *cannabidiol* is in second place. CBD accounts for up to 40 percent of the plant's extract.

Tetrahydrocannabinol (THC)

Cannabidiol (CBD)

CBD is a non-psychoactive compound found in cannabis. It was first discovered in 1940, but the chemical structure and stereochemistry were only identified in 1964.

Recent studies have shown how this compound can have great medicinal benefits. We have learned a lot about its positive effects, while its negative effects are zero.

Cannabinoids and how they work

A phytocannabinoid such as CBD or THC is a one of a class of diverse chemical compounds found in cannabis and hemp. These compounds act on cannabinoid receptors in cells and alter the release of neurotransmitters in the brain. THC, for example, alters the release of the neurotransmitter called *dopamine,* also known as the "feel good" chemical.

The human brain has multiple cannabinoid receptors. These are known as the *endocannabinoid* system. Two of them are currently specified as CB1 and CB2. These two cannabinoid receptors are also found in animals — mammals, birds, fish, and reptiles.

Cannabinoid receptors type 1

Cannabinoid receptors type 1 are primarily found in the brain, more specifically in the basal nuclei and the limbic system including the hippocampus. They are also found in the cerebellum and in both male and female reproductive systems. This accounts for a variety of effects once THC, for example, alters the release of neurotransmitters such as dopamine from cannabinoid receptors in the human brain.

Cannabinoid receptors type 2

Cannabinoid receptors type 2 are found mainly in our immune system, or in immune-derived cells, with the greatest density in the spleen. The peripheral nervous system runs through our body to connect our limbs and organs to the central nervous system which is found in the brain and spinal cord. So it acts as a line of communication between the brain and spinal cord and the rest of the body. CB2 receptors seem to be responsible for the anti-inflammatory effects and possibly other therapeutic effects of cannabis.

What does CBD do, exactly?

Cannabidiol is non-psychotropic, which means it has little affinity with the cannabinoid receptors type 1 and 2. But it acts indirectly as an antagonist towards THC and other cannabinoid agonists. This means that CBD counteracts the cognitive impairment associated with the use of cannabis. This tells us that CBD has medical potential without the psychoactive effects or "high" of the other compounds found in cannabis, such as THC. It means that CBD, or cannabidiol, has all the healthy benefits without the "buzz." So there is the opportunity for everyday medicinal use. As of right now, the effects of THC on one's mental health are still up for debate. Much research is still needed into its positive and negative effects and how it affects a person in the long term.

CBD does work on other receptors besides CB1 and CB2. It mainly affects receptors such as serotonin, adenosine, and vanilloid. The vanilloid receptor, or TRPV-1, has the function of detecting and regulating your body temperature and providing the sensation of scalding heat and pain. It is vanilloid that makes you sweat after eating hot peppers. CBD moderates these functions of the vanilloid receptor, revealing that it has anti-inflammatory qualities and can reduce pain.

But these are not the only roles that CBD plays inside the human body. Recent studies have shown that CBD is involved in the stimulation of the 5-HT1A serotonin receptor, which is known to have an anti-depressant effect. This receptor is common to a range of other processes such as appetite, pain perception, nausea, anxiety, and addiction mechanisms.

Last, but not least, CBD has been found to have a tendency to reduce the proliferation of cancerous cells and bone reabsorption by inhibiting GPR55 signalling. GPR55 is dominant inside the brain and has been associated with vital processes such as controlling blood pressure, modulating bone density, and preventing the proliferation of cancer cells.

We will talk more about this when we get to the health benefits of CBD and how you can use it as a medicine.

Medical uses and applications

CBD has the following medical properties that we currently know about:

-anti-emetic (reduces nausea and vomiting)

-anti-convulsant (suppresses seizure activity)

-anti-psychotic (combats psychosis disorders)

-anti-inflammatory (combats inflammatory disorders)

-anti-oxidant (combats neurodegenerative disorders

-anti-tumoral/anti-cancer (combats tumor and cancer cells)

-anxiolytic/anti-depressant (combats anxiety and depression disorders)

CBD as anti-convulsant

Studies over the last decade have shown CBD to have anti-seizure properties. It is reported that CBD has reduced the severity of seizures in animal models. In addition, there have been case studies on the effects of CBD on children with a drug-resistant type of epilepsy. All of this suggests there are great medicinal benefits from treatment with CBD.

CBD as anti-inflammatory

Some recent studies have shown CBD to have neuroprotective properties in cell cultures as well as in animal models with several neurodegenerative diseases. These diseases include Alzheimer's, multiple sclerosis (MS), Parkinson's, glutamate toxicity, and neurodegeneration (or brain damage caused by alcohol abuse.)

Numerous studies and recent clinical trials have shown that medicine containing CBD has successfully treated the spasticity associated with MS, or reduced its severity.

When it comes to Parkinson's disease, CBD has much to offer patients. CBD has shown it can improve the complex sleep behaviors associated with the rapid eye movement disorder. It can promptly reduce the symptoms of this disorder and help to improve sleep quality. It is safe to say that treatment with CBD has significantly improved the quality of life for scores of patients suffering from Parkinson's disease.

CBD as anti-tumoral/anti-cancer

There have been countless positive results from treating cancer patients with cannabinoids. Marijuana and cannabinoids have helped cancer patients to maintain a good appetite and to reduce their pain and sleeping problems. There are also positive signs that CBD has anti-tumor effects. Recently, several pre-clinical reports have shown that CBD reduced cell viability, increased cancer cell death and decreased tumor growth in cell structures and animal models. These effects may be due to CBD's anti-oxidant and anti-inflammatory properties. However, the effects of CBD on human cancer patients still need to be studied. Multiple industry-sponsored clinical trials are now underway to test the efficacy of CBD in human cancer patients.

With such great potential in the treatment of cancer patients, it is safe to say that CBD needs to be better acknowledged in the world of medicine, so we can get the best of what it can offer.

CBD as anxiolytic/anti-depressant

It is no secret that cannabis has the potential to induce acute psychotic episodes at high doses under certain circumstances. Several studies have suggested that using marijuana brings an increased risk of chronic psychosis to individuals with specific genetic risk factors. Research through studies and clinical trials has suggested that THC can cause these effects. It has also been suggested that CBD can act as an anti-psychotic and mitigate them. There have been a few small-scale clinical trials in recent years in which patients with psychotic symptoms were treated with CBD, including case reports of patients with schizophrenia, but the results were mixed. There was a small case study of Parkinson's patients with psychosis, which reported positive results for treatment with CBD. A small randomized clinical trial reported clinical improvement for patients with schizophrenia who took CBD over a certain period. Large randomized clinical trials would be needed to fully evaluate the therapeutic potential of CBD for patients with schizophrenia, bipolar disorder and other forms of psychosis.

CBD has shown in recent studies that it can reduce anxiety and stress, lowering both the behavioural and physiological (e.g., heart rate) measures of stress and anxiety in animal models. In addition, research through small human laboratory and clinical trials has shown CBD to be beneficial and efficient. The reports from those trials showed that CBD could reduce stress and fear in patients with social anxiety, when they were given a stressful public speaking task. In a laboratory protocol designed to model post-traumatic stress disorders, CBD improved "consolidation of extinction learning." In other words, patients were able to forget traumatic memories. The anxiety-reducing effects of CBD appear to be the result of altering the serotonin receptor 1 signalling, although more research is needed to fully understand this mechanism.

How you can use CBD

We have outlined what CBD does, how cannabidiol has great medicinal potential and how, backed by research and reports, CBD can work on different conditions, disorders and diseases. Now we would like to explain how CBD products are produced and applied to our daily lives. The most common form in which CBD is found is CBD hemp oil, but there are has many alternative forms such as pure concentrates, edibles, topicals and tinctures. End products range from pure CBD live resin, which has been derived directly from the plant, to special ointments and edible products such as CBD chocolate bars. These are sold throughout the United States and Europe by various online stores, homeopathic apothecaries, pharmacies, dispensaries and as a prescription drug on medical advice from a doctor, depending on where we live.

Cannabis, however, is a personalized medicine. The right dosage and regimen of treatment will depend on the individual and their condition. To achieve the maximum medical benefit from cannabis, be sure to choose cannabis products that include both CBD and THC because these two compounds complement each other and provide the best medical and therapeutic effects. The key factor in determining the right dosage of CBD-rich medicine is your sensitivity to THC. There are many who enjoy the high that THC in cannabis provides, and they can consume reasonable doses of any cannabis product without feeling too high or uncomfortable. But it is possible that you might find the effects of THC unpleasant. As we explained earlier, CBD can counteract its intoxicating effects. Obtaining the right balance between THC and CBD levels is your first step to getting effective treatment with cannabis products.

If you suffer from spasms, anxiety, depression, or pediatric seizure disorders, you may find initially that you get the best results from a moderate dose of a CBD-dominant product (a CBD/THC ratio of more than 10:1). But treating your condition or disease with a product that has a low level of THC, while not intoxicating, is not always the best option for treatment. Sometimes a combination of CBD and THC will have a greater medical effect on a wide range of conditions than CBD or THC alone.

For cancer, neurological diseases, and many other ailments and conditions, patients may benefit from a balanced ratio of CBD and THC. Extensive clinical research has shown how a 1:1 CBD/THC ratio is effective for neuropathic pain.

Your medical use of cannabis should be approached carefully, for optimal results. It can be a step-by-step process; in which you try to get the best possible ratio of THC/CBD in your medicine that will fit your condition. This gives you the option of starting with small doses of a non-intoxicating CBD-rich cannabis product. You observe the results and gradually try to increase the amount of THC. Simply put, the goal is to self-administer consistent, measurable doses of CBD medicine that include as much THC as you are comfortable dealing with.

Dosing with CBD oil

Brands of CBD oil tend to be confusing for consumers because they all have different standards of consumption and dosing. Many of these brands recommend way too much as a "serving" and others recommend too little. Personally, I would recommend starting with 25mg of CBD twice a day.

I also recommend you try increasing your dosage every three to four weeks by 25mg until your symptoms are relieved. You will need to decrease the amount of CBD if there is any worsening of your symptoms. For medical use, concentrations of CBD oils, extracts and concentrates may vary between preparations, ranging from one milligram per dose to hundreds of milligrams. This makes it easy for you to get the dosages you need in a form you find easy to use.

To increase appetite in cancer patients: 2.5 milligrams of THC taken orally, with or without one milligram of CBD, for six weeks.

To treat chronic pain: 2.5-20 milligrams of CBD, taken orally for an average of 25 days.

To treat epilepsy: 200-300 milligrams of CBD, taken orally and daily for up to 4.5 months.

To treat movement problems associated with Huntington's disease: 10 milligrams of CBD per kilogram of body weight, taken orally and daily for six weeks.

To treat sleep disorders: 40-160 mg of CBD taken orally.

To treat multiple sclerosis symptoms: Cannabis plant extracts containing 2.5-120 milligrams of a THC-CBD combination, taken orally and daily for 2-15 weeks. A mouth spray might contain 2.7 milligrams of THC and 2.5 milligrams of CBD at doses of 2.5-120 milligrams for up to eight weeks. Patients typically use eight sprays within any three hours, with a maximum of 48 sprays in any 24-hour period.

To treat schizophrenia: 40 to 1,280 milligrams of CBD, taken orally and daily for up to four weeks.

To treat glaucoma: a single CBD dose of 20-40 milligrams, placed under the tongue. Doses greater than 40 mg may actually increase eye pressure.

There is no established lethal CBD dose, but I urge you to read the product inserts carefully, to ensure you are taking the right amount of CBD. Discuss with your medical practitioner any questions or concerns.

How is CBD hemp oil used to create CBD products?

Companies, gardens and farms which grow cannabis for the production of CBD hemp oil have seasonal harvests of their high-CBD / low-THC strains. They will put their harvested buds and plant materials through a specialized, solvent-free extraction process to yield a hemp oil with a high concentration of cannabidiol. This pure hemp extract then has to be tested for safety, quality, and cannabinoid content before it gets processed in CBD products or hits the shelves directly as a concentrate. When it comes to CBD products in the states where cannabis has yet to be legalized, and medical use is restricted, your only option is to import it. The use of CBD is legal, but if you want to make it yourself you will have to derive it from industrial-grade hemp, and that process might *not* be legal—depending on whom you ask at the Drug Enforcement Association (DEA.) This makes CBD expensive in states where importing it is your only option, so be sure to support legalization if you think this needs to be changed.

Making your own CBD oil

This is a vital message to everyone who is considering using this method to extract their own CBD. As you are working with alcohol as a solvent, it is of utmost importance that you are aware of your surroundings concerning open fires, smoking stoves. and other situations that could mean potential harm and the risk of catching fire!

Before you start, measure the amount of CBD contained.

The safest way to measure how many milligrams of CBD your CBD extract contains is to have it lab tested, but that option is not always available. So here is a simple trick if you are obliged to measure it yourself. Understand that this method of measuring will not be the most accurate, but it will help to indicate purity and dosage, starting out with the plant material.

If you are not using cannabis for recreational purposes, I would recommend you use only buds that are grown for consumers for medical use, from certified dispensaries and farms. This means you're getting buds that are lab-tested for their THC/CBD levels, and you know what percentage of CBD and THC each gram of cannabis contains.

For CBD oil extraction, if you have the choice between several different strains with tested THC/CBD levels, you will want to pick those strains with high CBD levels and low THC levels. For people who are completely new to this, I need to explain that THC and CBD components are assessed at different levels. One to five percent THC is considered to be a low level of THC for a strain, while one to five percent CBD is fairly high. So at the high end of THC levels, you should be looking at 15 to 25 percent of THC per gram, whereas strains with a high CBD level are around 14 to 15 percent CBD. New strains of medical marijuana can be created by growing buds with higher THC/CBD levels.

For a good CBD oil extract, you should be looking for a CBD strain that has been tested with high levels of CBD, ranging from 5 to15 percent, while THC should remain at 5 percent, and preferably lower. If you are growing marijuana yourself, the THC/CBD levels should be provided with the seeds, if you're getting them from a professional cannabis seed company, since they offer a great variety of high CBD/low THC level strains. So you can choose the seeds that fit your requirements for medical marijuana. If you prefer a different balance of compounds (for example, if you want a high THC/very low CBD oil for daily use, with the uplifting and energizing effects of THC) the same rules of measurement are applied.

It all comes down to this: one percent of a single gram is 10 milligrams, so if you have a strain that contains 15 percent THC and 2 percent CBD, you are looking at 150 milligrams of THC and 20 milligrams of CBD. This is the way to measure the buds you are using if they are lab-tested and THC/CBD levels are provided.

If this is not the situation, and you didn't grow the buds yourself or have no way of ever testing them, you can't say anything about them. You can only speculate what the THC and CBD levels might be from the effects of using this cannabis. It's generally true that strains containing high THC and very low to almost zero CBD tend to produce a positive, uplifting and energizing effect. But they can also produce anxiety. Unknown strains, or cannabis purchased illegally with higher CBD levels (at the very rare maximum of 5 percent CBD per gram) usually get you stoned. These strains will relax you, sedate you, and give you a couch lock. They are a good antidote for stress and anxiety.

On the street it is almost impossible to encounter a pure CBD strain as a recreational drug, as the effects are strictly medical and won't get you high. Those 5 to 15 percent CBD /and 5 percent and lower THC strains will not make you feel high or stoned as the CBD completely counters the psychoactive effect provided by the small amount of THC. The best way to get those strains is to visit your local dispensary or grow them yourself.

Personally, I don't ever recommend buying marijuana illegally, because it usually hasn't been tested. There is the risk that such cannabis contains pesticides or powders such as calcium, milk powder and other materials to improve its weight. There is also a chance that glass-like, glossy chemicals such as hairspray or simply glass powder have been used to make it appear like a densely THC-covered nug or bud. With your illegally-purchased and untested cannabis, there is the risk it could be contaminated with PCP or other chemical drugs to improve its effects, which makes it potentially dangerous! This has absolutely nothing to do with the plant itself, but it is one of the dark sides of the drug business and an urgent reason for legalization! Remind yourself that this part of the business is still illegal, and vendors usually have no concern for users as long as there is money to be made.

Measuring the ingredients of cannabis oil

Here is where it gets a little harder to get exact measurements on your own. If you can possibly get your oil lab-tested I urge you to do so, since the following method is not always accurate. The larger the quantity of oil and cannabis used, the easier it becomes to measure the level of THC and CBD, given that you have the right information. You will need to apply the same formula to calculate CBD, but the amounts are more easily tested when they are larger.

So, for example, if you took a pound or 453 grams of lab-tested cannabis buds with 9.5 percent THC and 15.9 percent CBD, you would, technically, have 43.035 milligrams of THC (there is 95mg of THC in a gram so 95 x 453:1000 = 43.035 milligrams of THC in pound of buds.) The same principle applies to calculating the amount of CBD, where you take the 159 mg of CBD in a gram and multiply that by the amount of cannabis. So if you take 453 grams and divide the outcome by 1000, you would be looking at 72.027 milligram of CBD in a pound of buds tested at 9.5 percent THC and 15.9 percent CBD. Now that you know this, you're looking a potential 100 percent pure return in oil that should be 114.052 milligram.

This would be extraction done to perfection, but this is nearly impossible to achieve without proper experience and knowledge.

As you will be using cheesecloth to strain the plant material and raw bud to make this oil, you will have plant residue left in your oil which will bring the concentration down. However, I have seen, tested and used some very good home-made cannabis oils produced by this method, that were lab-tested at a level of 70 to 95 percent purity.

So now you know what to look for when you're making your own cannabis oil and want to measure the amounts of THC and CBD contained in it. But you want these measurements to be exact. For example: you have tested your product and are looking at 85 percent pure with 50 percent CBD and 35 percent THC in 100 grams of cannabis oil. This means you have about 15 grams of plant residue in your oil, but the oil itself is potent and of high quality. If you know your math and can use the metric system, this is will be easy to calculate, assuming you have been provided with the right information about the cannabis you're using.

In one of my upcoming books I will go into the world of cannabis extracts and concentrates in depth, as this is one of my passions and my field of expertise.

So how do you make the oil?

This is an easy way to extract cannabis oil using grain alcohol. This process will yield you about two to four grams of extremely potent, medicinal-grade CBD oil that is suitable for ingestion. After you've had a few practice runs, the entire process for small-batch edible oil production should take you about an hour, including around thirty minutes of cooking time. Grain alcohol is the solvent that is least likely to leave impurities or residue in the final product.

Supplies needed

One ounce of dried, ground-up bud material or two to three ounces of ground, dried trim/shake

One gallon of solvent (grain alcohol or other high-proof alcohol—never use rubbing alcohol)

Medium-sized mixing bowl (glass or ceramic is best)

Strainer (A cheesecloth/stainless steel kitchen sieve combo, or muslin bags, grain-steeping bags or even clean stockings/nylons)

Catchment container

Double boiler or bain-marie

Kitchen utensils (large wooden spoon, silicon spatula, plastic syringe for dosage and dispensing of oil, funnel)

Procedure

1. Get organized. Prepare your space, arrange your necessary equipment, find a level working area and make sure it is clean and set up before starting.

2. Place the ground-up cannabis material in the mixing bowl, leaving some space for the solvent. Find a larger bowl before proceeding further, if necessary.

3. Completely cover the plant material with the alcohol, adding about an extra inch of solvent above the top of the plant matter.

4. Using the wooden spoon, stir the cannabis material within the solvent for about three minutes. This enables the resin glands to dissolve into the solvent. Ensure the plant matter is thoroughly saturated and has had a chance to expel its resin content.

5. Place a straining bag or sieve into the catchment container. Pour the dark green liquid from the mixing bowl into the bag or sieve. Allow the liquid to be filtered completely as it goes into the container. Gently massage the bag in order to squeeze out as much liquid as possible.

Note: At this point you could repeat the previous four steps in order to extract as much resin as possible into the solvent. This second wash should remove most of the remaining resin.

6. Pour the strained liquid into the double boiler or bain-marie. You can place a smaller cooking pot inside the bigger one, so that the water in the bottom pot prevents the top pot from overheating or cooking too quickly. Fill the bottom of the double boiler or bottom pot with an appropriate amount of water. If your alcohol-resin solution doesn't all fit in the top of the double boiler or cooking pot, you can keep refilling the

pot as you boil down the CBD oil, eventually processing all of the rinse liquid.

7. Place the double boiler on high heat until the liquid begins to bubble, which is actually the alcohol evaporating. When it reaches the bubbling stage, turn off the burner. The residual heat of the water bath will continue to heat the mixture, allowing the alcohol to evaporate.

8. If the mixture stops bubbling, you may need to turn the heat back on, once or twice more. The evaporation usually takes between fifteen and twenty-five minutes to complete.

Note: The mixture should continue bubbling throughout the evaporation process. As the alcohol level decreases, so will the number of bubbles. It helps to mix the solution with the silicon spatula occasionally, scraping the sides of the pan.

9. Don't let the mixture get too hot, as this will damage the cannabinoids and compromise potency and flavour When the mixture is still runny but has stopped bubbling, turn the heat back on low until the mixture has begun bubbling again. Then turn off the heat. Continue stirring, which will allow even more alcohol to evaporate.

10. The oil is done when it has reached a thick, tar-like consistency and no longer bubbles. Since it continues to thicken as it cools, it is important to transfer the oil into storage or dosage containers at this point.

11. Slowly draw the CBD oil into the plastic syringes. As you reach the bottom of the pan, this will become more difficult, which is normal. Transfer any remaining amounts into small, air-tight containers. Aside from squeezing out small doses from the syringe, a toothpick can be used to apportion dosages.

Note: If a topical application is preferred, simply combine the CBD oil with olive or coconut oil while it is still warm. This also decreases the potency, stretching out the dosages for cash-strapped or less experienced users.

Topical and edible recipes made with CBD oil

The possibilities with CBD oil are almost endless but we'd like to provide you with two common recipes in which you can use your cannabidiol extract. We'll show you how CBD oil is used in a DIY topical hand balm and in classic, home-made CBD cookies.

CBD topical hand balm

Enthusiasts swear by CBD balm to treat all manner of ailments, including conditions such as rheumatoid arthritis, lupus, dermatitis and psoriasis. When properly prepared, topical cannabis balm can have analgesic, relaxing, anti-inflammatory, decongestant and regenerative benefits. Such balm preparations have existed in the human pharmacopeia for thousands of years.

Ingredients:

-½ ounce of cannabis with high CBD levels

-½ cup of Shea butter, coconut oil or beeswax (a combination of the three works best and is highly recommended)

Instructions:

1.Place the oils in a glass or ceramic mixing bowl. If you are using a combination, use a wooden spoon and mix them well.

2.Put a large pot on the stove and fill it halfway (or less) with water.

3.When the water is hot but not boiling, put the mixing bowl in the pot. Be sure no water gets inside the bowl.

4.When the oils have liquefied and are well blended, add your cannabis.

5.Continue to gently simmer, stirring every few minutes, for about 45 minutes. The longer it simmers, the more potent your salve will be.

6.Strain the salve through cheesecloth into another glass container. Squeeze the cloth to get out every drop you can from the cannabis.

7.Allow the salve mixture to cool completely before using.

*Once it has cooled, you can use a spoon or spatula to transfer it to a different container if you like. If stored in a cool, dark place, your balm will keep for about two months.

Note: Adding some beeswax to your oil will help to make your hand balm firmer and more stable. Using only beeswax will leave you with a hard substance which can be used as a lip balm but be sure, if you don't want that, to add at least one other type of oil to the mix.

You can also add almond oil or grape seed oil for a smooth, non-greasy balm. If you would like to have a sweet-smelling balm, add a dozen or so drops of the essential oil of your choice. Mix them in with the other oils you have chosen.

CBD cookies

If you love cooking and getting creative in the kitchen, this might be your thing. When we showed you how to extract CBD oil from cannabis plant materials, we said you could infuse this oil with either butter or coconut and olive oil. These are the ingredients that make your CBD-infused oil edible, and create many possibilities for original home cooking. In every recipe where butter or oil is called for, you can use your CBD-infused butter or oil. Below is a recipe:

Ingredients:

-2 ½ cups of flour, plus more for rolling

-1 cup of sugar

-1 cup of CBD-infused butter or coconut oil

-1 egg

-1 teaspoon of baking powder

-1 teaspoon of vanilla

-1 teaspoon of salt

Optional: powdered sugar and milk, for frosting.

For less potent cookies, switch out any portion of the CBD-infused butter and replace this with standard butter, as desired.

Instructions:

1.Beat your CBD-infused butter or coconut oil, sugar, eggs and vanilla in a large bowl on medium speed until the ingredients are thoroughly combined.

2.In a separate bowl mix the dry ingredients.

3.Add the dry ingredients to your CBD-infused butter mixture, a little at a time, stirring until all the ingredients are incorporated.

4.Cover the dough and refrigerate it for an hour or longer.

5.Preheat the oven to 375°F. or 180°C.

6.Roll out the dough on a generously floured surface to about one-third of an inch thick. Cut the cookies with a tumbler to press out some perfect circles. Transfer to ungreased baking sheets.

7.Bake for 10-12 minutes or until lightly golden.

8.Remove from the oven, transfer to a cooling rack, and let cool completely before frosting.

*To frost: combine powdered sugar with milk and stir until the desired consistency is reached. Then add food colouring as desired.

Yield: about 18 cookies.

Bonus reminder

Don't forget to grab your copy of 'The best DIY THC & CBD recipes to prepare at home' Go to: http://eepurl.com/cxpVZf

Subscribe to the HMPL Publishing newsletter, and we'll give you our free THC & CBD recipes to prepare at home book for free.

All you have to do is enter your email address to get instant access.

We don't like spam and understand you don't like spam either. We'll email you no more than 2 times per week.

To subscribe, Go to: http://eepurl.com/cxpVZf

You can also follow us on Facebook;
https://www.facebook.com/HMPLpublishing

Thank you

Finally, if you enjoyed this book, then I'd like to ask you for a small favour. Would you be kind enough to leave an honest review for this book on Amazon? It'd be greatly appreciated by both the future reader and me!

You can find the book in the Amazon store.

Did you discover any grammar mistakes, confusing explanations or wrongful information? Don't hesitate to send us an email! You can reach us at hmpl.publishers@gmail.com. We promise to get back at you as soon as time allows us. If this book requires a revision, we'll send you the updated ebook for free after the revised book is available.

Supportive research papers

Below is a list of all the titles used in the research for this book. You may look them up by searching the full title on Google, as most of them are publicly available.

Borgelt et al. *The pharmacologic and clinical effects of medical cannabis. Pharmacotherapy,* 2013.

Usar-Poli et al. *Distinct Effects of Δ9-Tetrahydrocannabinol and Cannabidiol on Neural Activation During Emotional Processing. Arch Gen Psychiatry,* 2009.

Jones et al. *Cannabidiol exerts anti-convulsant effects in animal models of temporal lobe and partial seizures. Seizure,* 2012.

Consroe P and Wolkin A. *Cannabidiol--antiepileptic drug comparisons and interactions in experimentally induced seizures in rats. J Pharmacol Exp Ther.* 1977 – Apr. 2011

Gloss and Vickrey B. *Cannabinoids for epilepsy. Cochrane Database,* 2014.

Iuvone et al. *Neuroprotective effect of cannabidiol, a non-psychoactive component from Cannabis sativa, on beta-amyloid-induced toxicity in PC12 cells. J Neurochem.,* 2004

Hampson et al. *Cannabidiol and (-)Delta9-tetrahydrocannabinol are neuroprotective antioxidants. Proceedings of the National Academy of Science, USA*, 1998.

Russo EB. *Cannabinoids in the management of difficult to treat pain. Therapeutics and Clinical Risk Management,* 2008.

Iskedjian et al. *Meta-analysis of cannabis-based treatments for neuropathic and multiple sclerosis-related pain. Curr Med Res Opin. 23(1):17-24* (2007).

Portenoy et al. *Nabiximols for opioid-treated cancer patients with poorly-controlled chronic pain: a randomized, placebo-controlled, graded-dose trial. J Pain.* 2012, May 13.

McAllister et al. *The Antitumor Activity of Plant-Derived Non-Psychoactive Cannabinoids. J Neuroimmune Pharmacol.* 2015.

Wilkinson et al. *Impact of Cannabis Use on the Development of Psychotic Disorders. Curr Addict Rep.* 2014.

Iseger and Bossong. *A systematic review of the antipsychotic properties of cannabidiol in humans,* 2015.

Guimaraes et al. *Antianxiety effect of cannabidiol in the elevated plus-maze. Psychopharmacology,* 1990.

Bergamaschi et al. *Cannabidiol reduces the anxiety induced by simulated public speaking in treatment-naive social phobia patients. Neuropsychopharmacology,* 2011.